Fitness For Life

Life's Health

www.LosingBellyFatMission.com

Contents

Intro

Dieting for life is a never ending struggle for many. However, dieting should be looked at as a way of life and not so much as an ongoing struggle. We should consume food that will enable us to lose weight or maintain a healthy body weight based on age, height, bone size amongst other important healthy weight indicators. It is important to maintain a healthy weight for yourself and your love ones. The list of healthy weight benefits are huge. Being overweight will put you at risk for many health risk factors including heart disease, hypertension and stroke. It's wise to get on a healthy diet plan and maintain it for life. Check out more tips at www.LosingBellyFatMission.com and transform your life.

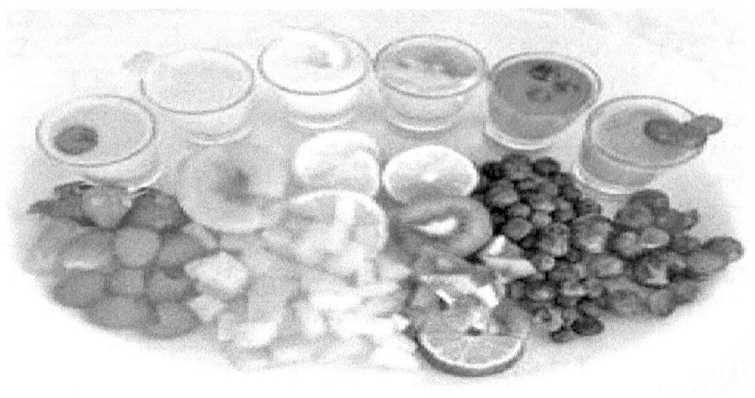

Sleep Can Contribute To Weight Loss

Dieters may make goals to start eating and living more healthy at any time. Although, knowing what techniques help in eliminating excess pounds as well as hindering diseases can make setting a goal easier. Thus, what exactly are these healthy ways to lose weight to assist with hindering illnesses? A great technique to reduce unwanted pounds is eating lots of vitamins, antioxidants and minerals. Antioxidants, minerals and vitamins aid with reducing excessive body weight because these items assist in keeping food cravings under control. Managing hunger leads to smaller amounts of products desired. Not as many food items desired leads to eliminating unwanted body weight. Consequently, dietary habits rich in minerals, vitamins and antioxidants are beneficial in getting rid of excessive pounds. Products loaded with antioxidants, minerals and vitamins that might want to be incorporated within every individual's diet plan include yams, bok choy and raspberries. In addition to aiding in losing unwanted fat, products rich in vitamins, minerals and antioxidants help prevent health problems. Vitamins, antioxidants and minerals strengthen the immune system. When the immune system is enhanced then the body is strong. As a consequence, chance for diseases like multiple sclerosis, viral communicable diseases and macular degeneration will be reduced. As a consequence, vitamins, minerals and antioxidants come into play for sustaining optimum health as well as body weight. An additional way in decreasing excess fat is getting adequate rest. Do not underestimate the benefits for obtaining plenty of rest. Research has proven a link amongst hormones and sleep which impact eating behaviors. If sleep deprived hormone that controls feelings of hunger is increased where hormone for sensing fullness decreases. Consequently, dieters experience an increase desire to consume food products and not sensing fullness. Additionally, individuals that lack sleep usually want mostly high calorie salty, starchy and sweet foods to snack on. Each of those items result in extra weight. Thus, obtaining enough sleep nightly is among the healthy ways to lose weight everyone should include. Besides aiding with reducing extra body weight, plenty of sleep helps prevent medical problems through keeping immunity raised. Sleep deficiency has been associated with a weakened immunity, anxiety and depression. Additionally, while sleeping a human body repairs abnormal cells from ultraviolet rays, stress and toxins. Consequently, try and obtain a minimum of seven to nine hours a night. To keep immunity increased will be beneficial for getting rid of extra pounds in addition to thwarting medical conditions. Comprehending particular food products in addition to getting sufficient quantities of sleep every night help in getting rid of extra pounds and hindering health conditions will be significant.

Cleanse Your Body With The Lemonade Diet

Size matters. Big or small, the body has been the point of concern for man and woman. An ounce of excess fat and you can see people working out till they get rid of it. But where is the time for today's world to go to a gym and work out a toned body, every day. Walking is one of the best methods of exercise, but what use is walking down polluted roads filled with corrupted oxygen and gray concrete woods. A balanced, fresh food diet is what is needed to have a healthy, clean body. The lemonade diet also known as the master cleanser, helps you to lose weight and cleanse your body organs of all impurities. It is a cleansing diet. Like every fruit juice diet, it is a fresh diet and short term. You need to follow the diet plan closely for at most a month to see its cleaning effects. More than weight loss, what a lemonade diet does is get rid off all the toxic substances hidden in various corners of your body and in the process remove the unnecessary fat as well. The lemonade diet came into existence through Stanley Burroughs in the magazine, The Master Cleanser. This original diet plan has been revised and modified by expert dietitians like Peter Glickman. The plan is to drink only lemonade for 10 to 40 days, supplemented only by raw vegetables and other dietary foods. This consists of freshly squeezed lemon juice, pure water, B graded maple syrup and cayenne pepper. Along with this, you need to drink, every morning, salt water flush and also a laxative tea every evening. Peppermint tea can also be added to the diet. As the diet closes to an end, it is important that you do not start eating normal food suddenly. You need to slow down the process starting with fresh raw vegetables and fruits and also cooked vegetable soups. The lemonade diet should be ended very slowly, and not in an abrupt manner. The only concern about the effectiveness of this diet plan is that it is deficient in the necessary nutrients needed by the body. As the body gets cleansed from its impurities you may experience short spans of nausea, vomiting and headaches. It is important that you follow your medical advisor's word while taking up this diet plan. Mostly 10 days are quite sufficient to feel the effect, but go with your physician's advice. The lemonade diet has been proved to be a god way to cleanse your body, and although it is difficult to live by only fluids and liquids for more than a week, it is effective.

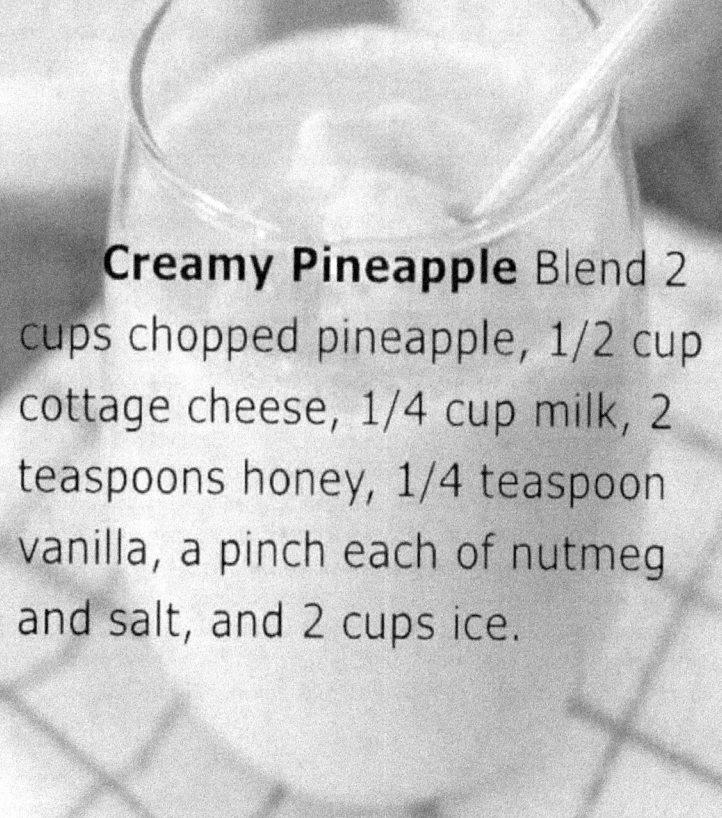

Creamy Pineapple Blend 2 cups chopped pineapple, 1/2 cup cottage cheese, 1/4 cup milk, 2 teaspoons honey, 1/4 teaspoon vanilla, a pinch each of nutmeg and salt, and 2 cups ice.

Low Carb Diet – You've Got To Be Kidding

Here is the problem with this crap about following a low carb diet program. To begin with, if you want to turn people off fast tell them they are going to have to drastically reduce the carbs they consume. That ought to do it, don't you think? But wait, then tell them they are going to have to "count" all the grams of carbohydrates and protein they eat. That should really get 'em going. But why couldn't you just tell it like it is? That in order to get healthy and maintain a healthy weight, you are going to have to quit eating carbohydrates that turn to blood sugar so fast that it screws up your insulin levels... and replace those with fresh fruits and vegetables like you know you should be eating in the first place? Then you could also remind them that insulin is a hormone and when it gets out of whack, other hormones get out of whack too, which compromises the immune system especially, as well as other vital systems in your body and whammo... you got a real mess going on. High Glycemic Carbohydrates Cause Exaggerated Insulin Levels I mean, most folks know that sweet cakes and candy, donuts and cookies, white bread, dinner rolls, etc. turn to blood sugar way faster than fresh fruits, vegetables, salads and whole grain breads, right? Well it just stands to reason that if those "bad" carbs turn to sugar a lot faster than "good" carbs do and cause your insulin levels to get out of whack, then before too long you're going to be in big trouble if you keep pigging out on that bad carbohydrate crap. Well, that doesn't mean that you necessarily have to cut down on carbs, does it? It just means that you have to cut down on junk carbs that are going to give you heart disease, diabetes, cancer or maybe even all three combined, right? But, then you're going to have to replace the "bad" carbs with good carbs and believe me, you're not going to be able to eat enough good carbs to ever do your body any harm. The best low carb diet program is the one that has you eating more carbs than you ever dreamed you could eat. And not just rabbit food either, but high quality, highly nutritious and appetizing "good" carbs, of which there are plenty available. The kind of carbs that when you eat them - the last thing on your mind is chasing it down with junk carbs. And we all know what "junk carbs" are, don't we? Low Glycemic Carbs Break Down To Glucose Slowly The best low carb diet plan is the plan that separates the good carbs, (low glycemic carbs), from the bad carbs, (high glycemic carbohydrates). You see, a good diet that will help you to live a healthier, happier life isn't one that makes you "cut-down" on anything. It is a diet that encourages you to eat more of the healthy food you should be eating and less, (way, way less) of the bad food you have known since you were a kid that you should not be eating. Whether it is carbohydrates, fats or protein, there is food that is good for you and food that is bad for you. You can call it a low carb diet program, a glycemic index diet plan, or just what it is; a good wholesome common sense way of eating. Either way, you can lose weight and be in the best shape of your life simply by having the discipline to eat like you know you should, or better yet... like your grandma and grandpa said that you should eat. It just takes a little common sense, a little planning, (that is where a program might come in handy), and a little bit of discipline to have the health you've always thought you should have.

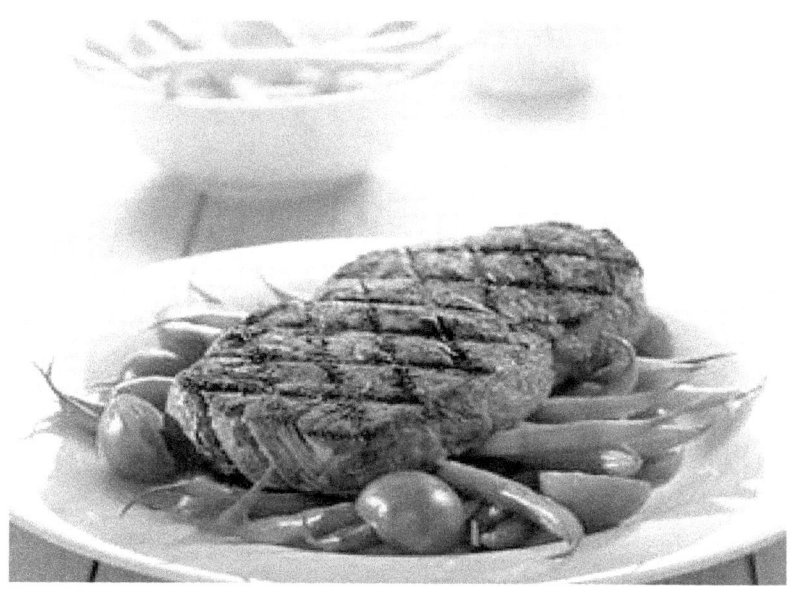

3 Easy and Natural Weight Loss Techniques – Lose Weight Ultra Fast

Problems are always a hindrance in every task that we do in every day of our lives. People always seek solution to lessen or eliminate these problems. One of these problems is how to lose weight as quickly as possible. In today's modern world, many techniques are developed through technology in order to solve existing problems as efficient as possible. As technology progress so thus techniques on how to lose weight progresses. Advances in herbal medication showed commendable results in losing weight. Consumption of natural herbal medicines, such as tea, is the popular choice. Tea is convenient in a way that it is easy to buy, easy to make, easy to prepare, and easy to consume. Herbal tea can be prepared anywhere whether you are at home, at your office, or can be ordered at any cafe near you. Tea can be prepared either hot or cold, your choice at your convenience. When tea is ingested into your system, nutrition goes directly into your bloodstream which account for the faster result. Another technique developed is the application of herbal injections or patches. This is a new and improved way to deliver natural herbal medicines into our system for a quick result. Patients who request this kind of medication can be done and performed by holistic doctors. Doctors then inject herbal medication directly into their system. Another way is the use of herbal patches. Just like nicotine patches, application of herbal weight loss patches are done on the skin. When patches are applied on skin, it is absorbed through the dermis of the skin and goes directly into the bloodstream. By the use of this technique, you can achieve incredible result without the hassle of remembering to take a pill several times a day. The third technique is the use of dietary herbal pills. This is widely known and still a viable option for a faster weight loss. Herbal dietary pills contains natural ingredients that help speed up metabolism, provide extra energy and burn fat that which accounts for faster weight loss. Any of these methods can be use for a faster result in losing weight. You can choose any of these methods depending on what your lifestyle is. However, every method has a proper procedure and proper personnel concerned for certain application. Always remember to follow directions and seek professional help before using weight loss technique of your choice.

Weight Loss Success – This is The Missing Link

If you're one of the millions who have struggled with weight loss, despite eating a healthy diet and exercising, then undetected food intolerance could be the missing link which can explain why your efforts fail. The good news is that you can do something about it. Many published studies confirm this viewpoint and explain why food intolerance can result in weight gain and obesity. Pelchats study in 2002 states that "It is well-known that individuals crave the foods to which they are intolerant and develop an addictive type relationship with particular foods". Sugar from foods like chocolate and alcohol can trigger the release of endorphins, the body's natural, powerful painkillers. The digestion of food proteins such as casein (dairy) and gluten (wheat) can stimulate the production of exorphins - opium like substances that are very similar to endorphins and attach to the same receptor sites. Over time these pleasurable brain chemicals can exert an addictive, drug-like effect similar to that produced by heroin and morphine that can be followed by withdrawal symptoms (such as cravings, overeating, weight gain, mood swings and guilt) if these foods are avoided. Does this sound familiar? When you have been over-eating certain foods that you are intolerant to, it is because your body is driving to maintain an opiate level, not necessarily to get high, but to avoid the dreadful feeling of withdrawal. It is not because you have no self-control. So give yourself a break. Medical researchers from Dubai reported in the Middle East Journal of Family Medicine that patients unable to achieve goal weight loss by calorie restriction alone were significantly aided in their attempts when they avoided foods that had been shown in a unique lab test to excite their immune system (Deutsch, 2009). In the 12 week study, the 27 patients underwent a single treatment: avoidance of foods that they were intolerant to. The foods were different for each individual. The results showed an average weight loss of approximately 37 pounds, an average drop of 6 points of BMI and an average decrease of 30% of body fat. Deutsch points out that hidden food intolerances or sensitivities are unique to each individual and can result in an inability to lose weight. We already know that food intolerances can cause people to crave the foods to which they are intolerant. Obese people can testify to the overwhelming power of food intolerance cravings. The obese person has no idea that his daily food cravings or eating habits can be due to a physiological need to stop withdrawal symptoms. It is possible to become intolerant to many foods, although there are foods that are more likely than others because we tend to eat them most often. Think about wheat which most people consume at least 5 or 6 times a day - wheat cereals, sandwiches, snack crackers, muffins, pasta, pizza, wraps and biscuits. If someone's addicted to coffee they may not necessarily get fat. If you are addicted to sugar or wheat, you may be running around with chocolate or breakfast bars in your pocket to satisfy your cravings. If you're intolerant to dairy and wheat, that might explain your unstoppable craving for pizza! What is most important is it is extremely difficult for food intolerant individuals to lose weight unless they ultimately gain control of their food intolerances. They must identify the food culprits, follow an elimination diet for at least 8 weeks and ensure the food intolerance is healed by making some small lifestyle changes and taking some supplements. Food intolerance can be cured and only then will people see real and sustained results with weight loss. In a Baylor Medical college study for the link between food intolerance and weight gain, 98% of subjects also displayed significantly improved body composition and/or scale weight following a food elimination diet within 4 weeks. A matched control group that followed calorie restriction alone actually became fatter. Deutsch (2009) claims that chronic inflammation, caused primarily by exposure to foods you are intolerant to, is at the root of metabolic problems like obesity. Food intolerance rates are rising to epidemic proportions with some studies saying up to 70% of us will suffer from one. The reason for rising rates comes back to lifestyle choices: eating processed, chemical-rich foods, too much alcohol and stress, exposure to toxins and chemicals in our environment and overuse of drugs like pain killers, antibiotics and the contraceptive pill. These choices cause the gut to become damaged or 'leaky' which leads to food intolerance. Left untreated for years, you can become intolerant to healthy foods too, like broccoli and pineapple. So if you think you fall into this category, there are 3 easy steps to follow to ensure you have sustained weight loss success. Do a food intolerance test which can be found online or from a nutritionist Eliminate and cure the food intolerance by strictly avoiding your problem foods and healing your leaky gut using supplementation Re-introduce the problem foods in a controlled manner to ensure the intolerance has healed Then you can follow your healthy eating and exercise plan and this time your body and metabolism will be working with you, not against you, to cut the fat storage. Given that food intolerance is not a subject many doctors know much about - there's no drug to prescribe to cure it - it's no real surprise that this 'missing link' has been overlooked. Who's doing the big research and getting it into the media anyway? Certainly not the pharmaceutical companies, the diet food companies or any other part of this dieting industry. It's down to you but at least this time there's no fad diet, just a sensible 3 step plan to success. Disclaimer: The use of this information is not a substitute for health advice. Please consult your doctor, pharmacist or health care provider for specific medical advice. The information should be used in conjunction with guidance from your medical practitioner as he/she will be aware of your unique personal medical history.

Food And Drinks To Avoided on a Diet For Pregnancy

If you are one of those expectant mothers who are now conscious of what they eat, a diet plan for pregnancy can come in handy. Through this, you can keep track of what you are eating and you can be assured that you get the right amount of vitamins and nutrients if you follow your diet plan. In devising one, you must know what foods to eat and what to avoid. Because a developing baby is delicate and vulnerable, you have to be mindful of what you eat so as not to harm your baby. However, you have to pay close attention to the food that you consume. There might be times that you eat certain meat or fish that you think you are already getting the proper nutrients when in fact you are not. Choosing the correct type of food plays an important role in your diet. Fish should be included in a diet plan for pregnancy because it contains omega 3 fatty acids and iron beneficial for pregnant mothers and growing babies. However, there are certain types of fish that you should avoid due to high content of mercury and other pollutants. Swordfish, king mackerel, tilefish and shark are those types of fish that you should exclude from your diet. Sushi, oysters and raw fish should also be avoided because they may have harmful bacteria. On the other hand, fish such as mahi mahi and wild salmon are good options. Milk and dairy products are also included in the diet plan. However, some products should be avoided because of harmful bacteria. Listeria is a harmful bacterium that can sometimes be found in food items. Soft cheeses stored in the refrigerator can contain Listeria so you should avoid eating this. Hot dogs and cold cuts should also be avoided because of possible Listeria contamination. Another harmful bacterium found in food is salmonella. Raw eggs should be avoided as these may contain this bacterium. It is also found in meat that is not well cooked. In order to avoid this, beef and other meats should be cooked well, that is, until no pinkish color can be seen. Alcohol is a big no-no in a diet plan for pregnancy. It affects the baby's brain and overall growth. Birth defects can happen because of alcohol so there should be complete avoidance. Coffee intake on the other hand is still debatable up to date. More than a cup of coffee per day may harm the baby. Some believe that caffeine intake of less than a cup per day is not harmful although studies show that there Is minimal risk to the fetus. It is best that you avoid it as well. Instead of these drinks, fruit juices and milk are greatly suggested. Also avoid processed foods and unhealthy fats and oils so that you will have a healthy body and a healthy baby.

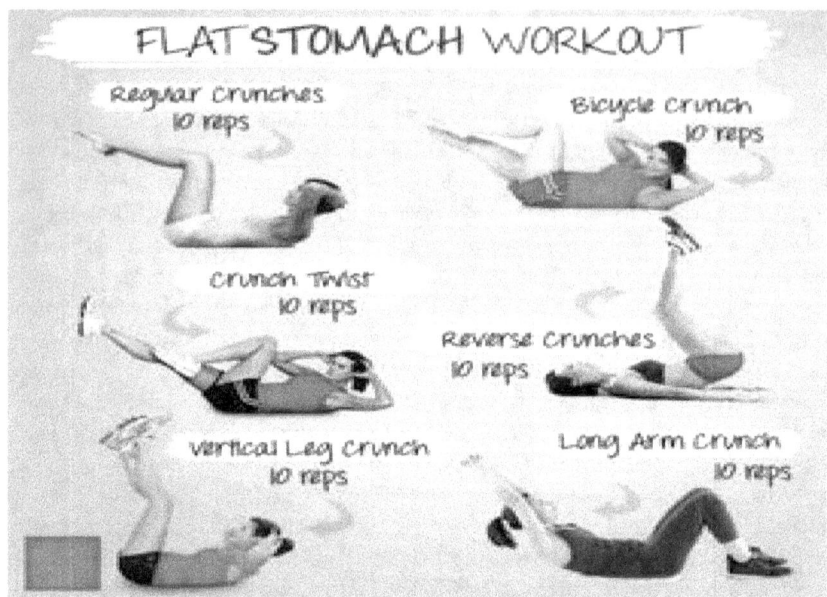

Resistance Training Diet – The 5 Things You Mustn't Neglect To Achieve Results Fast

Nutrition is the most vital component of building muscle, but is sometimes overlooked. The reality is that, you might not be able to establish new muscle tissue if your body does not get the right nutrients. An important thing to keep in mind is that you need to consume more calories than what you would normally use daily. Although, this doesn't mean that you should lean towards eating junk food. Having a better grasp of nutrition will be necessary in order to plan meals well and ultimately build a strong physique. The Rules of Good Nutrition 1) Having a diet which is well balanced The three crucial nutrients that you need to have in your bodybuilding diet plan include protein, carbs, and fat. As a general rule of thumb, your daily calorie intake should come from 60% carbs, 30% protein, and 10% fat. Remember to include a number of food items within your diet from each of the food groups. Dairy products such as milk and cheese are nutrient-dense, although it will be best to limit their intake as they are high in saturated fat and simple sugar. Vegetables and fruits on the other hand are packed with essential nutrients, and you'll require about four to six servings of these each day. And, also beans, nuts, poultry and meats are rich in protein and are great sources of foods for building new muscle. Carb rich grains are yet another thing worth including in your body building diet plan. While, junk food still needs to be reasonably limited. 2) Have six small meals with protein eating more often in smaller serving sizes works best so that your body can take in all the calories you eat. Instead of having large meals for breakfast, lunch and dinner, split them up into six smaller portioned meals spread across the day. Where, Protein needs to be be added to each meal. 3) Drink lots of fresh water a daily aim of half a gallon p/day is what you will want. A bodybuilding diet plan requires adequate water. Not only is your body made up of 70% water but it is crucial for digestion. Remember to drink around about one liter of water as you workout. This will provide enough hydration for the body. 4) Take multi-vitamin or mineral supplements You may wish to include some essential nutrients to what you are already eating via supplements. But, realize that fruit and veggies can provide enough vitamins and minerals without the need for supplements. It's only really when there are not any fresh products available. 5) Purchase and store good food If you aren't used to purchasing fresh food, change your habit today and include more of them in your bodybuilding diet plan. When you buy fresh meat, choose leaner cuts with less amount of fat. You can also purchase organ meat like heart and liver which are excellent sources of protein, vitamins, and minerals. If you're not going to use the meat within two days, freeze it. Label the meat so that you will know the how old it is. When buying poultry, buy large birds, and freeze if you are not planning to use it immediately. Buy fresh and firm fish with shiny and bright skin. Refrigerate them and consume within two days. When it comes to fruits and vegetables, buy firm ones in different colors. You can refrigerate the vegetables for up to a week. But store your fruits in room temperature. Plans for Bodybuilding Diet Here is a sample food list which you can follow to build your muscle mass. * Ideas for breakfast A cup of porridge Omelet made from egg-whites * Ideas for lunch Meat sandwich with salad stir fry beef Roast pork 21.5 pounds * Ideas for snacks Nuts Carrot sticks or cherry tomatoes To sum it up, having a good bodybuilding diet plan will keep your muscle-building goals on track and also helps to avoid junk food cravings.

7 Bad Habits That Would Spoil Your Diet Plan

There are too many temptations will stand in your way when you are setting a goal to regulate your eating patterns. Whether it's a birthday party at the office or it's your family day out for dinner. Clearly these kind of situations are very challenging for you. Who would stand for not participating tasting the chocolate fountain, some sweets, or a T-Bone that being presented on the table in front of you. Without you knowing it, you are messing your own diet program. Now, if you want to succeed it, you have to know some other bad habits that could spoiled your diet plan so that your diet program would not obstructed. 1. Leftovers You may feel guilty to yourself or to your friends and family if you don't finish up your foods that you have ordered at some restaurant or dining place. But this feeling of responsible to finish up your meal may result in: your waist will become more and more stretchy. The solution to this kind of situation is, Put only a small amount of food on your plate. If portions of food that you ordered is too big, ask some of your food to be wrapped. It's easy, right? 2. Too paranoid of unhealthy foods Allow yourself to occasionally enjoy your favorite foods. If you put too much restriction to yourself for not enjoying your favorite meal for once in a while, you will have this urge inside to eat more than usual. You can just observe first at the grocery store or at some food chain restaurant the packaging label so you can learn the nutritional information, such as "low fat" or "sugar free". If you do that and have to right information about the foods you are about to eat, you will think twice to eat more than usual. 3.Wanting what others have Maybe you have a friend that have a thin body even though she/he eating some junk foods every time you guys hang out together. But, you can't compare yourself to her/him. Do you know why? It's because there are people that were born with fast metabolism. Genetic factors and certain medical conditions affect the metabolism. Also, consider this: are you also diligently working out like your friend? Learn what makes your friends can stay lean. After that, you can just enjoy every meal without guilt. 4. Not a cooking person You probably said to yourself that you're a lousy cook or maybe you don't like the mess that you gonna make at the kitchen during and after cooking, so you decide to take delivery order or eating outside, which can lead you to eat some fatty or over calorie foods. If you cook, you can control the nutrition or the ingredients of your food, and then you can keep a small portion of your food in the fridge to eat later. Another good thing is you also don't have to cook something else when you're hungry during midnight. 5. Lack of sleep The more you reduce the hours you sleep, your body will increasingly lack leptin, a hormone that helps you lose weight. When you are sleep-deprived, hormone ghrelin, which stimulates appetite, higher rise. That is why people tend to feel hungry or have this urge of craving when they stay up all night. You have to try to sleep for at least 7 hours a day. If you can't have sleep 7 hours during the night, try to take a short nap on the next day. 6. Skipping breakfast If you skip your breakfast, you will tend to feel very hungry and the sandwich you brought from home for you lunch is not gonna be enough. Or if you having lunch with some friends from your office at some restaurant, you will eat anything on the menu. If you used to skip breakfast every morning, your blood sugar will drop very fast and you will feel very hungry during lunch time. 7. You think you have a slow metabolism, so you just eat a little You need at least 1500 calories every day. However, if metabolism is very slow, you may be able to consume 1,200 calories per day, supplemented with a multivitamin and two calcium pills 500 mg. Also, make sure you keep nutritious food choices (with vegetables, fruits, grains, meat, and healthy fats). For a while, forget the old junk food. Try also to eat foods in smaller portions but more frequently throughout the day. This will prevent your blood sugar to drop dramatically. Click To Continue.

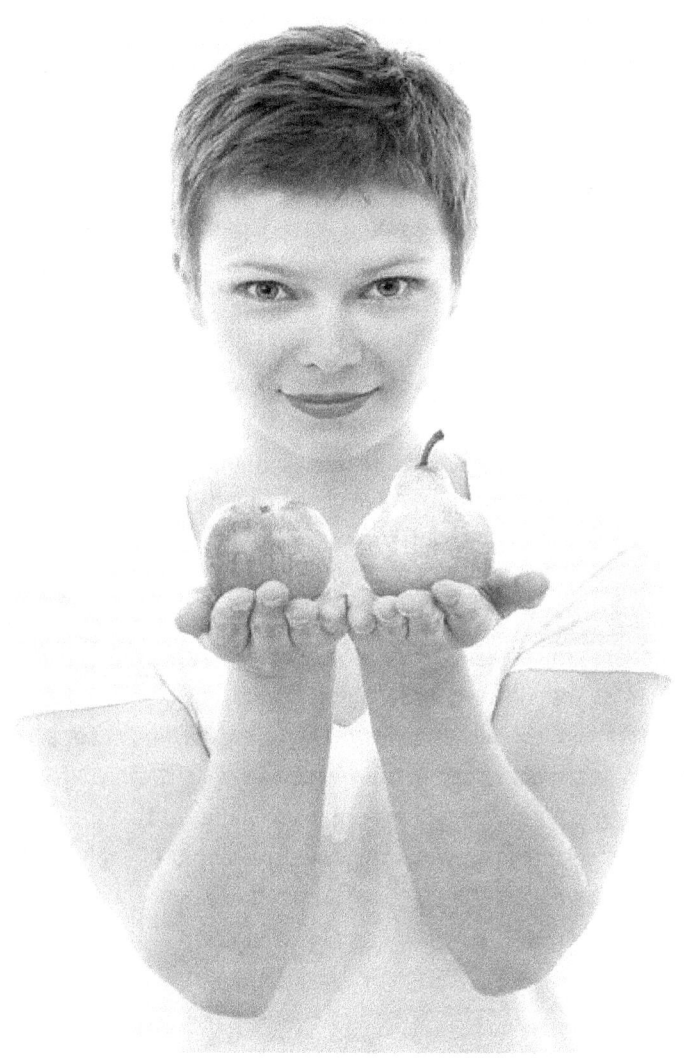

One of the newest hypes in dieting is the so-called "Negative Calorie Diet Plans," which, some claim, can make you lose extremely large amounts of weight (as much as 14lbs per week). But what exactly are these plans? Do they work? Are they even safe? The principle behind negative-calorie diets, is that the dieter should eat mostly foods that provide lesser calories than the body consumes by processing such foods, but which can make you feel full. For instance, let's say you eat a meal that fills you up and provides a total of 100 calories, but your body will eventually burn 150 calories just by digesting and metabolizing this meal, so you actually lose 50 calories just by eating this meal. The type foods recommended for this diet are watery vegetables which are made mostly cellulose or fiber and which are rich in vitamins, minerals and water, and have very little nutritious value from carbs, proteins and especially from fats. Lettuce, tomato, broccoli and carrots would be good examples of these foods. The main idea would be to fill up as much as possible on these foods, so the body does not get the minimum caloric requirement to replace lost calories during the day, while the person does not feel hungry due to fasting. Even though in principle these diet plans might be effective in shedding relatively large amounts of weight quickly, they pose some serious dangers to the person's health, and might not actually produce the desired results.

Some of the most dangerous consequences of following a diet of this type could be loss of muscle mass, loss of bone tissue, damage to organs, diseases such as anemia, chronic joint pain, chronic fatigue, etc. On top of that, you might actually be keeping the fat, instead of losing it, while you actually slow down your metabolism. One of the biggest misconceptions in weight loss is that the more you cut down on calories, the faster you lose weight. What most people do not realize (and many fitness experts forget to tell you) is that when you drastically cut down on your caloric intake, your body goes into what is known as "starvation mode."

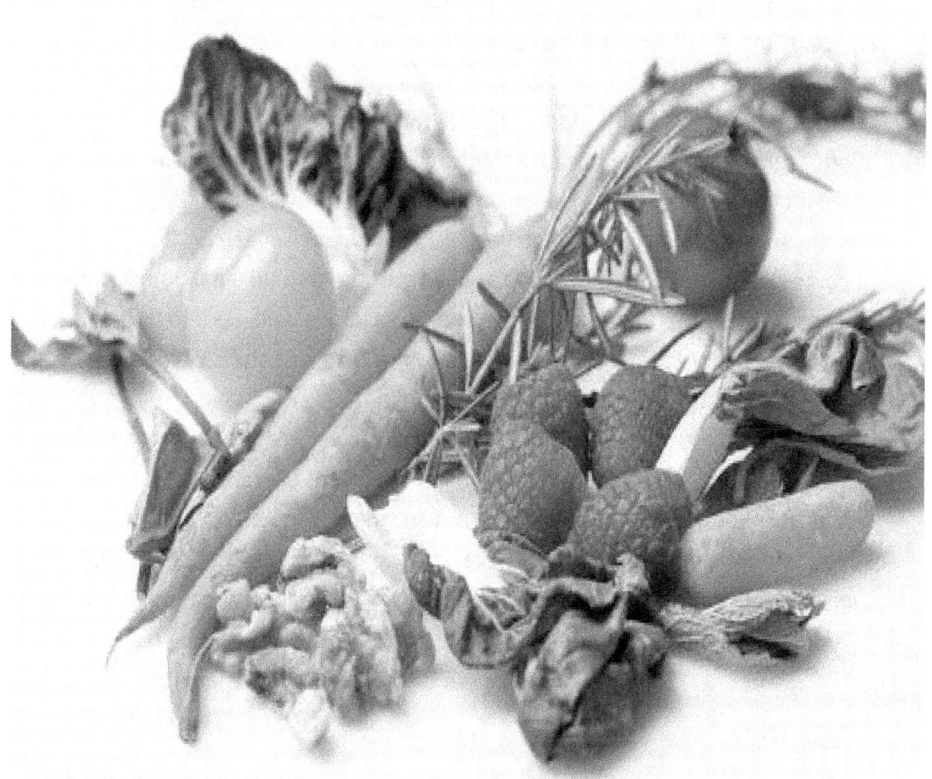

Simply put, when you cut down too much on calories, your body "thinks" there is not enough food available to survive and as a defense mechanism, it will try to save as much energy as possible by slowing down its metabolism. And guess, what is the last thing the body will use as an energy source? That's right: the fat. The main reason for this is that fats are the hardest nutrients to break down, while at the same time they have the largest caloric value (while 1g of carbs or proteins contains 4 calories, 1g of fat contains 9 calories, which is also the reason why fat is harder to burn). That is why it is not recommended to cut down too much on calories at once. So, even though the principles of a negative calorie diet plan might work in theory, they might end up being a disaster in the practice. However, it would be a great idea to consume these "negative calorie" foods to help with cravings, in between meals, or just to help you add bulk to your "real" meals. It is always very important to understand how your body works and what the medical implications are, before you decide to try any type of weight-loss or fitness program. This is why no fitness program is a good substitute for expert advice from a qualified physician or health professional. Remember that every day we hear of new programs and systems that promise us to lose weight, build muscle and look like Hollywood stars and, most of the time, we will never hear about them again, simply because they do not do what they promise to do. So, when it comes to losing weight, the most important advice I could give to you is this: If you want to achieve a goal, you MUST do your research on the topic, become familiar with the terminology and truly understand what you are facing. If you are truly serious about a goal you want to achieve, you need to understand every aspect about it and take the time and effort to research every aspect of it before you can achieve it. Even though some methods might work really well, you will still have to make an effort. And you should always consult with a qualified physician before you try a new fitness program. There are no such things as "Magical Solutions" to your problems, but solving them does not have to be an impossible task, either. As a matter of fact, it could become a lot easier than you think if you just have the right information.

Great Heathly Foods:

There are tons of food that are healthy for you, but you just have to choose the right ones and stick to it. When you do so you will be on healthy diet that make sense. You will also get to see some of the benefits of a heathy lifestyle in regards to all that comes with it. There is no way around living a healthy lifestyle. I'm not saying you can't have something that you really enjoy from time to time that might not be healthy, but you can't eat like that everyday and expect to be living on a clean diet. You have to take a break from garbage food, and focus on what makes more sense to consume regularly.

15 QUICK AND DELICIOUS
SEAFOOD RECIPES

Seafood Lovers Recipes

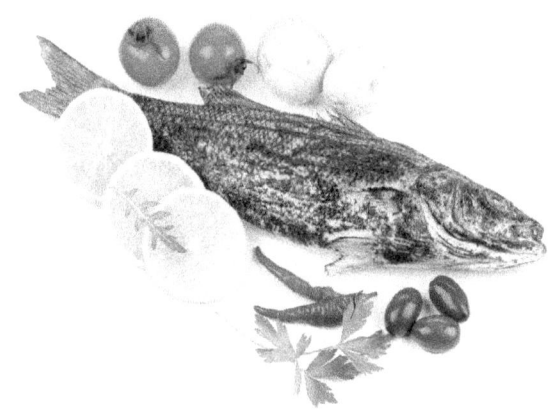

OSWIN DACOSTA

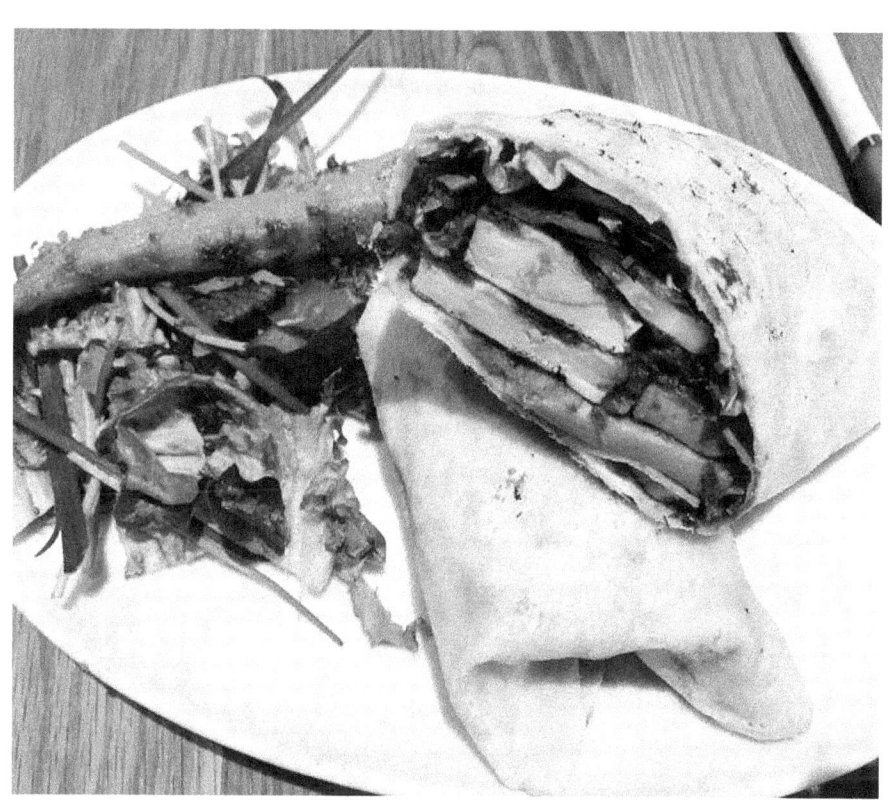

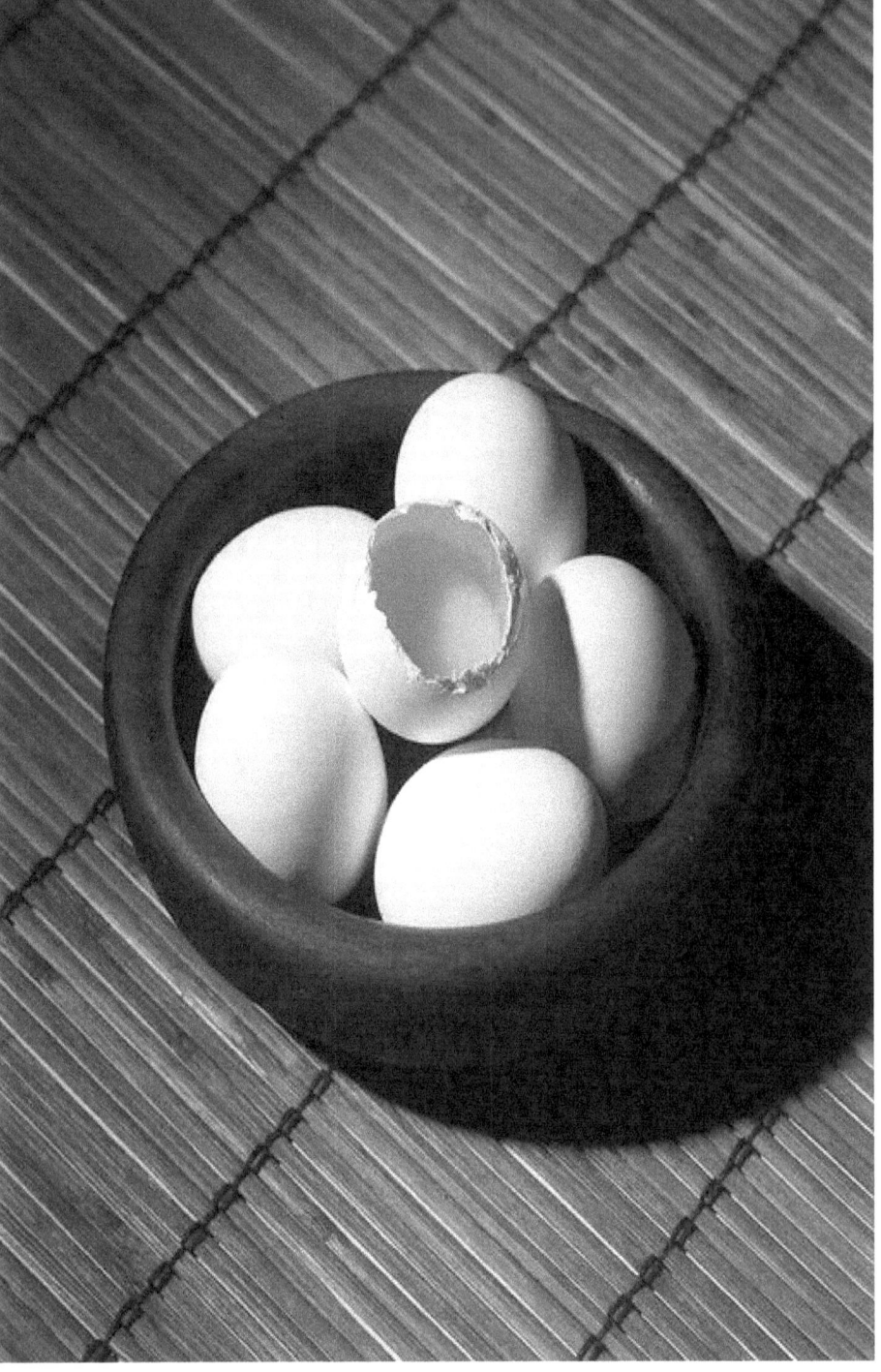

www.ingramcontent.com/pod-product-compliance
Lightning Source LLC
Chambersburg PA
CBHW072016280526
45788CB00005B/2063